Paleo Performance

Boost Your Fitness with Ancestral Nutrition

Table of Contents

Chapter 1. Introduction

Unveiling a game-changer in your fitness journey, our Special Report on 'Paleo Performance: Boost Your Fitness with Ancestral Nutrition' is dedicated to helping you unlock your optimum health and vitality! Harnessing the wisdom of our ancestors' dietary habits, this report draws exciting connections between nutrition and physical performance. Far from an ordinary guide, it marries ancient wisdom and modern scientific understanding in a dance of knowledge that might just be the missing link in your exercise routine. Unpack the transformative potential of Paleo nutrition with user-friendly, accessible research that could catapult your fitness to awe-inspiring heights. This unique ticket to your fitness aspirations is not just informative–it's positively thrilling! Get ready to prime your body the way nature intended and revolutionize your workouts forever. Purchase this special report today and take that exhilarating leap towards unbelievable physical achievements.

Chapter 2. The Fundamentals of Paleo Nutrition

Let's embark on this voyage of discovering the bedrock of Paleo nutrition, which blends the ancestral wisdom of hunter-gatherer diets with the advanced insights of recent nutrition science. This chapter will empower you with the knowledge you need to integrate this transformative dietary strategy into your everyday lifestyle effectively, enhancing your fitness performance.

2.1. Foundations of Paleo Diet

The Paleo diet, which is also referred to as the 'caveman diet', is rooted in mimicking the nutrition patterns of our Paleolithic ancestors, dating back to approximately 2.5 million to 10,000 years ago. Contrary to modern agricultural and dairy practices that have grown prominent in the contemporary age, the early human diet was confined to what could be hunted, fished, or gathered. Such foods included lean meats, fish, fruits, vegetables, nuts, and seeds. It's this simplistic, yet nutritionally-dense approach that the Paleo diet aims to encapsulate.

2.2. The Nutritional Profile of a Paleo Diet

A balanced Paleo diet incorporates a rich portfolio of nutrients that your body requires for optimum functionality. Though micronutrient content may vary based on specific meal composition, Paleo meals generally prioritize:

1. High protein intake: Lean meats, fish, and eggs are paramount in supplying essential amino acids, supporting muscle synthesis,

recovery, and overall body functions.

2. Healthy fats: The Paleo diet welcomes a selection of monounsaturated fats, polyunsaturated fats (particularly Omega-3 fatty acids), and saturated fats, predominately derived from nuts, seeds, fish, avocado, and virgin oils like olive and coconut oil.

3. Low-moderate carbohydrates: Paleo focuses on minimizing refined sugars and grains, favoring instead higher-fiber, lower-glycemic fruits, and vegetables.

4. Fiber: Whole fruits and vegetables, along with certain nuts and seeds, provide the necessary fiber, promoting healthy digestion and satiety.

5. Vitamins, minerals & antioxidants: By promoting a wide variety of colorful fruits and vegetables, the Paleo diet naturally supports an abundance of essential vitamins and minerals, as well as antioxidants, for optimal health and recovery.

By understanding these nutritional targets, it's possible to design satisfying, delicious Paleo meals that align with your fitness goals.

2.3. The Role of Processed Foods

In contrast to many contemporary diets, Paleo strongly discourages processed foods. High in artificial additives, refined sugars, and unhealthy fats, processed foods veer away from the 'whole food' ideology central to Paleo principles. Industrially processed foods often lack vital nutrients, are low in fiber, and high in sodium, contributing to inflammation and other health risks.

2.4. Foods To Embrace and Avoid

A simple rule of thumb in choosing Paleo-approved foods is asking the question, "Could a caveman eat this?" If the answer is no, it's probably not Paleo-friendly.

Consequently, your Paleo diet should include lean meats, fish, fruits, vegetables, nuts, and seeds—foods that in the past could be obtained by hunting and gathering. Conversely, avoid foods that became common when farming emerged about 10,000 years ago, such as dairy products, legumes, and grains.

Indeed, adhering to the Paleo diet means ditching modern, processed snacks and 'convenience foods' and replacing them with more wholesome, nutritionally-dense alternatives. Pre-packaged foods, sodas, cereals, and all forms of candy are examples of what to steer clear from.

2.5. Tailoring Paleo to Your Fitness Goals

The beauty of the Paleo diet is that, while it does set out some fundamental guidelines, it is highly adaptable to individual needs and goals. If your aim is to gain muscle mass, a higher intake of lean protein and healthy fats can support this pursuit. Conversely, if you're seeking weight loss, reducing carbohydrate intake and focusing more on high-fiber vegetables and lean meats may be more beneficial.

Whichever your fitness goal may be, it's important to remember that dietary changes should be complimented with an active lifestyle. Paleo wasn't merely a diet for our ancestors - it was their way of life.

In conclusion, the Paleo nutrition philosophy can act as a powerful catalyst for fitness improvement. By opting for ancestral dietary habits, we equip our bodies with the fuel they need for optimal functioning and resilience. Through Paleo's eye-opening approach, you will discover not just a diet, but a lifestyle rooted in health, vitality, and longevity—a passport to unparalleled fitness success, all through the nature-led wisdom of our ancestors.

Chapter 3. Understanding the Ancestral Connection: Nutrition and Fitness

Our physical fitness today is significantly defined by our nutrition. Intriguingly, a fresh lens into this relationship can be found in the ancient past. As a species, our nutritional past has shaped our beings - an idea that's grounded in the concept of evolutionary mismatch. Simply put, humans have not undergone any significant genetic change in the past 10,000 years, but our diet and lifestyle have drastically shifted, especially in the last century. The 'mismatch' between our genes and our current nutritional environment could be at the heart of modern health issues like obesity, heart disease, and diabetes.

3.1. The Evolutionary Narrative

To understand the impact this shift has had on human health, it's crucial to trace the journey of our ancestors from hunter-gatherers to today's society.

The Paleolithic Era, spanning nearly 2.6 million years, saw humanity in its most primitive stages. The human diet then was primarily composed of lean meat from wild animals, fruits, vegetables, nuts, and seeds, with little to no consumption of grains, dairy, or processed foods. This food selection was not out of choice but necessity, driven by the immediate environment and hunter-gatherer lifestyle.

As we journeyed into the Neolithic Era and agriculture was born, our nutritional landscape started shifting. Humans began growing crops and rearing livestock, drastically altering our dietary habits. This introduced grains and dairy into our regular diet. Dove-tailing this, was the industrial revolution that ushered in processed foods, sugars, and unhealthy fats.

However, our modern diet is at odds with our genes that have evolved over millions of years to function best on a diet rich in proteins, healthy fats, and low-glycemic carbs. This stark disconnect could explain the prevalence of nutritional and metabolic disorders we see today.

3.2. A Look At The Ancestral Plate

Our Paleolithic ancestors consumed a diet rich in macro and micronutrients, essential for their high-energy lifestyle. Let's look at what constituted an ancestral plate:

1. Lean Meats - Wild animals provided a rich source of protein. These proteins were not only essential for building and repairing muscles but also provided the body with essential amino acids, B-vitamins, iron, and zinc.

2. Fruits and Vegetables - These were rich sources of vitamins, fibre, and important minerals.

3. Nuts and Seeds - Apart from being a good source of protein, nuts and seeds were also rich in healthy fats and fibre.

4. Seafood - Where available, seafood was consumed. It provided a punch of omega-3 fatty acids, essential for cognitive function and cardiovascular health.

Note the obvious absence of dairy, grains, and legumes, staples of today's diets. Contrarily, the variety and high nutrient-density of the Paleolithic diet underpins the health, vitality and physical prowess of our ancestors.

3.3. Back To The Roots: Paleo Diet and Fitness

Modern fitness enthusiasts are rediscovering the secrets of our ancestors and applying them to athletic performance. The Paleo diet could be a vital tool for enhancing physical fitness by optimizing nutrition based on evolutionary biology. Here is how this connection manifests:

1. Higher Protein Intake - Essential for muscle recovery and growth. The Paleo diet places a strong emphasis on high-quality proteins that allow for better athletic performance.

2. Balanced Energy Consumption - Unlike modern diets high in carbohydrates, the Paleo diet relies more on fats and proteins for sustained energy, leading to better endurance and prevention of energy crashes typical of high-carb diets.

3. Anti-Inflammatory Benefits - The Paleo diet is rich in foods known for their anti-inflammatory properties, reducing the risk of injuries, hastening recovery, and improving overall fitness levels.

4. Micronutrients - The Paleo diet provides a range of essential vitamins and minerals, like iron, magnesium, and B-vitamins, that are critical for optimal physical performance.

5. Digestive Health - The gut plays a critical role in fitness. The Paleo diet is void of processed foods and sugars, leading to better gut health which in turn positively impacts energy levels and immune function.

Following the Paleo diet principles could bridge the evolutionary digestive gap and might lay the groundwork for improved physical performance.

3.4. The Caveats

While the Paleo diet is quite promising, it's important to acknowledge that it's not a one-size-fits-all solution. Genetic and individual variations affect how different individuals respond to different diets.

Also, critics argue that certain valuable food groups, such as whole grains and legumes, are eliminated in the Paleo diet. These foods do provide several nutritional benefits and may not necessarily be harmful if consumed in moderation.

3.5. Conclusion

While our diets may have evolved with our shifting ages and technologies, it appears that our genes haven't caught up. Reflecting upon our ancestral diet shines a new light on the nutrition-fitness link. The Paleo diet, harking back to our evolutionary past, has promising potential for modern fitness enthusiasts to meet their nutritional needs and perform at their peak. But, like all diets, it should be tailored to individual needs and health profiles. It's less about mimicry and more about understanding the wisdom of our ancestors and interpreting it in our modern context. By unlocking the secrets of our ancestral nutrition, we may just stumble upon an exhilarating new frontier in performance nutrition.

Chapter 4. Debunking Myths about the Paleo Diet

The Paleo diet, also referred to as the caveman or Stone Age diet, stems from the eating patterns of our ancient ancestors who lived during the Paleolithic era, a period lasting around 2.5 million years that ended about 10,000 years ago. The core concept of Paleo is to align your diet with the nutritional habits of pre-agricultural, hunter-gatherer ancestors who did not have access to modern grains, sugar, and processed food.

Despite its increasing popularity, the Paleo Diet remains cloaked in misconceptions. What follows is an exploration and clarification of several common misconceptions related to this diet.

4.1. Desolating the Dairy

A prevalent myth about the Paleo Diet is that all dairy is off-limits. It's easy to perceive why this notion exists: dairy foods weren't available during the Paleolithic era. However, Paleo is more flexible than you might think. Though it encourages avoiding processed dairy products like cheese spreads, some variants of the diet permit the inclusion of organic and grass-fed dairy items like ghee, butter, yogurt, and even certain types of cheese, due to their health benefits and high nutrient content. By this logic, if dairy isn't a problem for your body, there's no reason to exclude it outright.

4.2. Wholesale Rejection of Legumes and Grains

Another myth is that the Paleo Diet opposes all legumes and grains. The truth is a bit more nuanced. Paleo guidelines suggest avoiding grains and legumes because of the possible presence of anti-nutrients like phytates and lectins, which can interfere with nutrient absorption. However, methods like soaking, sprouting, or fermenting can reduce the amount of these anti-nutrients, making such foods more digestible and less likely to cause inflammation. Individuals who aren't sensitive, with a well-functioning digestive system, can consume responsibly-prepared grains and legumes under a modified Paleo diet.

4.3. The Supposition of High Protein

The Paleo diet is often mischaracterized as being super-high in protein. While protein is a critical part of the diet, it is not the only focus. The Paleo Diet also emphasizes the importance of maintaining a balanced ratio of macronutrients—carbohydrates, fats, and proteins. It recommends obtaining protein from varied sources, such as meat, seafood, eggs, and certain plant-based foods rather than relying on protein shakes or supplements.

4.4. Expensive Eating Does Not Equal Paleo Living

Another misconception about the Paleo Diet revolves around the expense. People often believe that Paleo eating is prohibitively costly because of its emphasis on organic produce and grass-fed or wild meats. However, it's possible to follow a budget-friendly Paleo lifestyle. Many Paleo followers advocate investing in high-quality proteins while supplementing with less expensive, seasonal, locally-sourced vegetables and fruits. Additionally, the potential long-term healthcare savings due to improved health can offset the cost.

4.5. Starving Over Starch

There's a common fallacy that the Paleo diet proposes no starch consumption. While it's true that Paleo encourages choosing vegetables and fruits over grain-based foods, that doesn't mean that starchy vegetables are out of the picture. Foods like sweet potatoes, yams, plantains, and others are often included, given their rich nutrient profiles and the sustained energy they provide.

4.6. Challenging the Cholesterol Concerns

Many people believe that the Paleo diet can inadvertently increase cholesterol levels due to high consumption of fats, particularly from meat. However, quality is just as important as quantity when it comes to dietary intake. Paleo emphasizes lean meats with reasonable fat content and encourages an abundance of fruits, vegetables, and healthy fats, which can all contribute to healthy cholesterol levels.

In conclusion, it's essential to gather accurate information and look beyond the common misinterpretations associated with the Paleo Diet. Every diet or lifestyle change should be adapted to suit individual needs and preferences. By debunking these myths, one can better understand the Paleo approach's core aspects and make an informed decision on whether this diet can help attain their health and fitness goals. The Paleo diet, when followed attentively, may prove to be an effective strategy for sustainable health and performance.

Chapter 5. Fit Like a Caveman: The Role of Paleo Nutrition in Physical Performance

The Paleo diet—also known as the caveman diet—has been gaining momentum in the fitness world as people have come to appreciate its potential merits. Inspired by our hunter-gatherer ancestors, this diet depends heavily on whole foods, namely lean meats, fish, fruits, vegetables, nuts, and seeds. This chapter delves deep into this primal way of eating and underscores how diet patterns, similar to those followed by our ancestors, could potentially revolutionize physical performance.

5.1. The Cornerstones of Paleo Nutrition

The Paleo diet encourages consumption of nutrient-dense foods that our bodies have evolved to process over millions of years. Essentially, it prompts you to eat the way our ancestors did before the advent of agriculture and mass food production.

The principal constituents of the Paleo diet include high-quality proteins (lean meats, fish, and poultry), carbohydrates from fruits and vegetables, healthy fats, and a modest amount of nuts and seeds. These ingredients provide an excellent mix of macronutrients—proteins, fats, and carbohydrates—alongside a host of essential vitamins and minerals.

5.2. Role of Protein in Physical Performance

Lean protein, a significant component of the Paleo diet, lays the foundation for heightened physical performance. When you engage in physical activity, your muscle fibers suffer microscopic damage, which is then repaired through protein synthesis to create stronger and larger muscles. A diet high in high-quality proteins provides all the essential amino acids necessary for effective muscle recovery and growth.

5.3. Healthy Fats and Energy Calibration

While the modern fitness industry often vilifies fats, the Paleo diet embraces healthy fats as indispensable. These healthy fats—monounsaturated and polyunsaturated fats—are sourced from foods like avocados, nuts, seeds, fish, and high-quality meat. They are essential for numerous bodily functions such as hormone production and inflammation control. In terms of performance, fats can also act as a robust and enduring energy source for long and intense workouts.

5.4. Carbohydrates: Fueling Performance

Contrary to popular belief, Paleo is not a low-carb diet but rather, it is a diet that highly advocates for complex carbohydrates. The diet is rich in fruits and vegetables, which provide the body the energy it needs to sustain exercise. These complex carbohydrates also ensure slow, steady, and long-lasting energy release to maintain stamina and vigor.

5.5. Micronutrients for Optimized Athletic Performance

It's not just the macronutrients that matter; the Paleo diet is also loaded with essential vitamins and minerals. A plethora of fruits, vegetables, lean meats, and fish in this diet provide a bounty of iron, zinc, potassium, magnesium, and vitamins, critical for energy production, efficient oxygen transportation, and enhanced immune function—factors significant for physical performance.

5.6. Paleo Nutrition and Hydration

Hydration plays a vital role in athletic performance and the Paleo diet, in no means, overlooks this aspect. Plenty of fruits and vegetables in the Paleo diet naturally supply the body with fluids. Moreover, the lack of processed and sugary foods that contribute to dehydration is another exceptional aspect of this nutritional approach.

5.7. The Mechanisms of Paleo Nutrition in Physical Performance

The standards of Paleo nutrition create a symbiotic relationship with physical performance. The emphasis on protein fosters muscle growth, repair, and recovery. The focus on complex carbohydrates afforded by fruits and vegetables ensures energy that's sustainable. Healthy fats support hormone function, which can impact performance. Micronutrients play their part in maintaining and enhancing various physiological processes for top-level performance.

5.8. The Benefits Beyond Physical Performance

A Paleo nutritional approach offers benefits beyond just improved physical performance. This diet is inherently anti-inflammatory, promotes optimal digestion, improves sleep, and stabilizes blood sugar—factors that, although indirectly, will impact physical performance over time.

In conclusion, a Paleo diet can be a game-changer for your fitness journey. With energy-packed nutrition, anti-inflammatory benefits, efficient digestion, and improved energy calibration, Paleo nutrition holds promise for those keen on making significant strides in their physical performance. In the next chapters, we'll delve further into specifics of how you can implement and personalize Paleo nutrition for your unique needs and health objectives.

Chapter 6. Boosting Your Workout Regime with Paleo

The Paleo diet, often referred to as the 'caveman' or 'stone age' diet, is centered around foods that our ancient ancestors are believed to have consumed. This includes meats, fish, vegetables, fruits, nuts, and seeds, making it a nutrient-dense, wholesome regime that continues to gain popularity among fitness enthusiasts for its natural, unprocessed approach.

6.1. Navigating the Paleo Way

Before adopting the Paleo diet into your workout regime, it's important to first integrate your understanding of what it means to 'go Paleo'. You're essentially working to consume foods that hunters and gatherers would have eaten during the Paleolithic era. While this includes a wide variety of lean meats, fish, fruits, vegetables, nuts and seeds, it restricts the intake of processed foods, grains and dairy products. The standard proposed ratio of a Paleo diet is roughly 55% of daily calories from seafood and lean meats, 15% from fresh fruits, and the remaining 30% from fresh/frozen vegetables.

6.2. From Cave to Gym: The Benefits

Science suggests that our bodies are designed to metabolically thrive on the types of foods that were available to our early ancestors. Consuming a pre-agricultural, hunter-gatherer diet can offer numerous health benefits, including higher protein intake, low-glycemic index, more fiber, more healthy fats, enhanced mineral and vitamin density, and greater balance in energy consumption. All of these factors aid in general physique and form the nutritional foundation that can enhance your workout potential drastically.

6.3. Structuring Your Paleo-Diet

Efficient planning can alleviate the hurdle of preparing meals. Paleo Breakfasts, for instance, can be composed of eggs cooked with assorted vegetables, slices of avocado, and a small portion of fruit. A post-workout lunch could be a filling salad packed with leafy greens, colorful veggies for vitamins and fiber, grilled chicken for protein, or salmon for omega-3 fatty acids. Dinners could be heavier on proteins, like roast beef or pork chops complemented by a mix of sautéed veggies. Snacks can be nuts and fruits.

6.4. Maximizing Workout Performance with Paleo

Studies suggest that the Paleo diet holds significant potential for improving workout performance. Its protein-dense nature aids in avoiding muscle catabolism (the breakdown of muscle fibers), while the healthy fats provide sustained energy. Furthermore, the anti-inflammatory components of the Paleo diet can help fasten recovery post-workout. With a Paleo diet like this, energy spikes and crashes associated with high-carb, low-fiber diets are diminished, and you can optimize your performance in the gym.

6.5. The Role of Protein and Natural Fat

In Paleo, protein and natural fat play crucial roles. Protein is essential for the growth and recovery of muscle tissue. Natural fats provide a long-lasting energy source, usually burnt during endurance workouts.

6.6. Carbohydrates in the Paleo Diet

Unlike modern diets that often include processed and refined grains, the Paleo diet simplifies the carbohydrate aspect. It promotes consumption of fruits and vegetables, which are natural, unrefined carbohydrates rich in fiber.

6.7. Transitioning: A Step-by-Step Guide

Transitioning to a Paleo diet might be challenging initially. Begin by replacing processed foods in your diet gradually with nutrient-rich alternatives, such as swapping processed meats for lean, organic cuts. Gradually increase the intake of fruits, vegetables and nuts instead of relying on grain-based foods.

6.8. Paleo Pitfalls

While the Paleo diet brings numerous benefits, certain pitfalls should be avoided. For instance, over-consumption of red meat can result in an increased cholesterol intake. Also, while the diet discourages grains, it's important to ensure that you receive enough fiber and other nutrients commonly consumed from whole grains.

6.9. Conclusion

In sum, the Paleo diet has the potential to drastically enhance workout performance by providing balanced nutrition, optimized energy usage, and faster recovery. Careful planning and adherence can help create a perfect synergy between your diet and exercise regime, taking your fitness aspirations to unparalleled levels. By incorporating Paleo principles, you're embracing an ancestral path that can lead to a significant transformation in your physical capabilities.

Chapter 7. The Power of Proteins: Meat and Seafood in the Paleo Diet

The importance of protein in human nutrition is undeniable. It is a cornerstone of all biological life, and for humans, it plays a key role in maintaining vitality, energy, and strength. Proteins, after all, are the building blocks of muscle tissues. But in the context of the Paleo diet, this macronutrient takes center stage as the power driver in transforming your physique and workout results.

7.1. Role of Protein in the Paleo Diet

The Paleo diet, also known as the caveman diet, promotes eating foods that our Stone Age ancestors would have had access to, including lean meats, fish, fruits, vegetables, nuts, and seeds. In a typical Paleo diet, the bulk of caloric intake – typically 20 to 35% – comes from protein.

One can understand the preferred status of protein in this dietary regimen from the standpoint of our ancestors. They didn't have easy access to agriculture, so their diet predominantly consisted of hunted food, rich in proteins. Moreover, considering their active lifestyle, proteins provided not only a stable energy source but also assisted in rapid recovery and growth of muscles.

7.2. Protein Sources in Paleo: Meat & Poultry

The Paleo diet encourages the consumption of free-range, organic, or grass-fed meats as they are more closely related to the nutritional profile of the game meat our ancestors consumed. Modern industrial meat is often full of antibiotics, hormones, and, in some instances, disease, which detracts from nutritional quality. Consuming these meats regularly can negatively impact our bodies causing inflammation and digestive issues, among other problems.

Beef, pork, lamb, chicken, turkey, and other game meats are good sources of protein, packed with essential amino acids that promote cell growth and repair. These meats also provide significant amounts of important micronutrients like iron, zinc, and vitamin B12.

7.3. Seafood: An Underestimated Protein Source

While meat holds a prominent space in the Paleo diet, seafood cannot be overlooked. Fish and shellfish are excellent protein sources with the added benefit of being lean and carrying important nutrients like Omega-3 fatty acids. These essential fats help fight inflammation, protect heart health, and can even enhance brain function.

Fish, particularly fatty fish like salmon, mackerel, and sardines, are the champions of Omega-3s. Shellfish, including clams, mussels, oysters, and scallops, also offer significant nutritional value, in addition to their high protein content. Not only do they provide Omega-3s, but they're also packed with important minerals like zinc and iodine, which support immune function, thyroid function, and overall metabolic health.

7.4. The Magic of Eggs

Although eggs are not strictly meat or seafood, they are a fantastic protein source that aligns with the principles of the Paleo diet. They are nutrient-dense, providing vitamins A, B, D, and E plus selenium and iodine. Eggs are often referred to as 'nature's multivitamin' due to their impressive nutritional profile.

Eggs, specifically yolks, are also rich in choline, a nutrient crucial for brain development and function. Many people, especially women of childbearing age, do not get enough choline in their diets, which makes eggs an excellent addition.

7.5. Protein: A Dietary Catalyst for Muscle Recovery and Growth

An essential component of your fitness journey, protein consumption, tied with regular exercise, fosters muscle recovery and growth. When you exercise, your muscles experience tiny tears; your body uses protein to repair and strengthen those tissues. Therefore, sufficient intake of protein can increase muscle mass, strength, and overall physical performance.

7.6. Benefits for Weight Loss

Multiple studies show that protein can be a game-changer when it comes to weight loss. High-protein foods require more calories to digest and metabolize, creating a thermal effect and stimulating weight loss. Protein also triggers the release of hormones like PYY and GLP-1, which indicate satiety and help control the appetite, leading to a lower caloric intake overall.

Chapter 8. Conclusion

The power of proteins, particularly from meat and seafood, is arguably one of the most important aspects of the Paleo diet. It isn't just about building muscles or reducing the waistline. It's about choosing nutrient-dense foods that come packed with proteins, essential amino acids, and other nutrients that your body needs for optimal function. Integrating high-quality proteins in your diet, supported by regular physical activity, can bring you closer to your fitness goals, creating a foundation of strength, vitality, and well-being. The Paleo diet isn't a trend or a quick fix; it's a lifestyle that honors the wisdom of our ancestors' eating habits and a path to long-term health.

Your fitness journey will always be personal and unique. However, armed with the knowledge you've gained from understanding the power of proteins, you can craft a Paleo diet that fuels your body, maximizes your workouts, and promotes holistic well-being. When it comes to the dance of your health and vitality, proteins are the rhythm that drives the music.

Chapter 9. Roots and Tubers: Unearthing the Plant Side of Paleo

The first footprints of humankind imprinted the soil in Africa, eons before the trappings of modern civilization, our ancestors had thrived and evolved by tuning their bodies to the land's offerings. Of several elements shaping our ancestor's dietary landscape, roots and tubers occupied a significant position. Foragers didn't merely subsist on these gifts of the Earth's belly; they thrived, setting the foundations for our species' impressive evolutionary journey.

9.1. The Allure of Ancestral Nosh

Our ancestors' plates buzzed with diversity that's seldom mirrored in our modern diets. As hunter-gatherers, they didn't rely on farming for sustenance, but foraged from the wild, hence the term 'wild food'. Roots and tubers were a part of this 'wild food'. Surprisingly dense in nutrients, these carried the powerful potential to buoy health and wellbeing. Equipped with protein, fiber, and complex carbohydrates, these humble-looking life forms were, in fact, a powerhouse of energy and nutrition. Through evolving research, we've come to uncover the surprising bounty that these tubers and roots packed.

9.2. Nurturing with Nutrients

Roots and tubers are an impressive source of nutrients, some of which may surprise the modern eater. They are filled with vitamins and minerals. Complex carbohydrates provide a steady energy stream, and fiber helps aid digestion and fosters good gut health. Probiotic properties in some roots and tubers support the microbiota, the collection of beneficial bacteria in our digestive systems.

Additionally, roots and tubers are low in fat and reasonably low in calories, making them a worthy part of a fitness-focused diet.

9.3. In the Heart of Paleo Performance

Tubers and roots have proven to be allies in the fitness journey. The energy-dense complex carbohydrates in these plants assist in steady energy release, perfect for long, strenuous workouts. The fiber fraction delays hunger pangs, helping to curb overeating. An added boon comes from their beneficial impact on gut health, pivotal for overall body vitality and immune resilience.

9.4. Power Plants: Famous Roots and Tubers

There's a dazzling variety of roots and tubers that were, and still are, a part of the human diet. Here are a few:

1. Sweet potato: Packed with fiber, vitamins, minerals, and antioxidants, sweet potatoes are a tuber possessing the power to support a strong body.

2. Cassava: High in resistant starch and a good source of Vitamin C, cassava flourishes in tropical climates.

3. Taro: Valued for its high potassium and fiber content, taro is a staple in several Asian cuisines.

4. Beets: Sporting a vibrant hue and rich taste, beets are an excellent source of folate, manganese, and other valuable micronutrients.

9.5. Beneficial Bounty: Health Impact of Roots and Tubers

Integrated well into a Paleo diet, these roots and tubers carry a profound potential for health enhancement. The nutrients nourish the body, and the gut-friendly properties can lead to better immune function and overall health. Whether you're looking for energy for your workouts or for fiber to help with weight management goals, roots and tubers can play pivotal roles in your Paleo performance, much as they did for our ancestors.

Unearthing this ancestral wisdom isn't just an exercise in nostalgia; it's a robust strategy for wellness. Indeed, by going 'back to the roots', we encounter a dietary approach that resonates with our physiology, promoting energy, vitality, and ultimate physical performance. The Paleo diet doesn't aim to replicate their lives but to inspire ours with lessons from their successful survival. Embrace these lessons to forge a unique path towards your fitness goals, wielding the proven power of roots and tubers in your wellness journey.

Chapter 10. Vitamins and Minerals: Pillars of Paleo

The strides that the Paleo diet offers in fitness transformation aren't limited to lean proteins and quality carbohydrates–vitamins and minerals play just as critical a role. These micronutrients, though they don't supply energy, are absolutely indispensable for countless physiological functions including metabolism, immunity, and, yes, physical performance.

A comprehensive understanding of which vitamins and minerals we should prioritise and why, goes miles in tailoring our Paleo practices and reaping their full benefits. Let's dive into each one's unique properties, natural sources, and necessity for our body's optimal functioning.

10.1. Role and Importance of Vitamins and Minerals

Vitamins and minerals are involved in every aspect of our physiological functioning. They help with energy production, immune function, blood clotting, bone health, and affect our overall physical performance. Although they are only needed in small amounts, the absence or lack of these nutrients can lead to significant health problems. Therefore, obtaining these micronutrients from our diet-instead of synthetic supplements-ensures that our body can absorb them in their most bioavailable form.

10.2. B Vitamins: The Vital Energy Catalysts

B vitamins play a critical role in your body, primarily by aiding in converting dietary energy into ATP (adenosine triphosphate), the form of energy your body utilises. The Paleo diet's richness in lean meats, vegetables, and fruits naturally provides a healthy supply of these vitamins.

- **B1 (Thiamine)**: Good sources include pork, fish, peas, and asparagus.
- **B2 (Riboflavin)**: Present in eggs, liver, and a variety of vegetables like spinach and broccoli.
- **B3 (Niacin)**: Chicken breasts, red meats, salmon, and fresh Tuna are rich in niacin.

10.3. Vitamin D: The Sunshine Vitamin

Vitamin D, central to bone and immune health, lets us absorb calcium and phosphorous. Though sunlight allows our skin to produce vitamin D, food sources like fatty fish, egg yolks and offal can be of immense value, particularly for those living in regions with less exposure to the sun.

10.4. Vitamin A: The Bio-Regulator

Vitamin A is key in maintaining healthy vision and regulating gene expression. The Paleo diet promotes nutrient-dense organ meats and leafy greens, both of which are abundant in vitamin A.

10.5. Vitamin C: The Immunity Booster

Vitamin C or ascorbic acid plays a major role in the synthesis of collagen, healing wounds, and enhancing iron absorption. Paleo-approved fruits and vegetables, such as citrus fruits, strawberries, and bell peppers, are excellent sources.

10.6. Essential Minerals and Their Food Sources

Minerals are also pivotal for maintaining optimal health. Some of the crucial minerals and their Paleo-friendly food sources are:

- **Iron**: Crucial for the formation of hemoglobin, iron comes aplenty in red meats, seafood, and spinach.

- **Zinc**: Involved in immune function, proteins and DNA synthesis, you can find zinc in oysters, beef, and almonds.

- **Magnesium**: This helps in regulating various biochemical reactions in the body, and one can acquire it from nuts, seeds, and green leafy vegetables.

- **Calcium**: Essential for bone and teeth health, it's abundant in dairy products, fish, and almonds.

10.7. Balancing Micronutrients for Optimal Health

Achieving just the right balance of these micronutrients can be tricky. It is important to learn to listen to our bodies and understand how different nutritional components interact with us individually. Additionally, some micronutrients, such as iron and calcium, can compete with each other for absorption, so they should not be consumed at the same time.

10.8. Incorporating Vitamins and Minerals into Your Diet

Despite being a no-grain diet, Paleo doesn't mean a lack of diversity. Getting a wide variety of whole foods is the golden rule and will provide a wide spectrum of these micronutrients. A typical day to incorporate all these elements might look something like:

Breakfast: Scrambled eggs with vegetables and a side of strawberries.

Lunch: Grilled chicken with a vibrant, leafy salad topped with almonds.

Dinner: Grilled salmon with a side of asparagus or broccoli.

10.9. Making Smart Choices

Adopting the Paleo diet isn't about blindly restricting food groups - it's about making smarter decisions about the food we consume. Keeping the emphasis on whole, nutrient-dense foods rich in essential vitamins and minerals is core to the Paleo principle. By doing so, you don't just fuel your body for the next workout, you nourish it for a lifetime of optimal functioning and wellness.

The Paleo diet provides a nutrient-rich framework that is particularly beneficial when it comes to the supply of essential vitamins and minerals. When properly followed, it can offer a variety of nutrients from natural and unprocessed sources. Embrace this wisdom of our ancestors and forge your path to improved health and fitness today.

Chapter 11. Case Studies: Real-Life Success Stories of Paleo Performance

The journey into health and fitness is not only about finding the right fuel for your body but also realizing that this pathway is not singular but varied. The Paleo diet's success stories abound with people who've transformed their physical abilities remarkably. Let us delve into some of these inspiring narratives that paint a vivid picture of gains realized through committed adoption of Paleo performance principles.

11.1. Maya's Meteoric Rise in Marathons

Maya, a marathon enthusiast from Boston, had hit a plateau with her running times. Despite rigorous training over two years, she was unable to break her personal best record. With the introduction of the Paleo diet, however, her story took a turn for the better.

Maya switched to a diet abundant in lean proteins, vegetables, and healthy fats, eliminating processed foods, dairy, and grains. Her daily nutrient intake primarily consisted of lean cuts of meat like chicken and turkey, a variety of colorful vegetables and fruits, and sources of healthy fats like avocados and nuts.

After two months, she noted a significant increase in her energy levels, which showed in her training. She saw her recovery times shorten, inflammation decrease, and her performance started to peak. Six months into her Paleo journey, Maya managed to smash her previous best by 15 minutes, a feat she attributed to her newfound dietary habits. This case is not only a testament to her personal commitment but also to the potent impact nutrition can have on athletic performance.

11.2. Ethan's Epic Transformation Through CrossFit

Ethan, a 30 year-old Texas native, turned to CrossFit to shed some extra pounds and build muscle. After six months of training with negligible results, he began exploring dietary alternatives.

Ethan's Paleo journey began by giving up his staple diet of cereals, pasta, and high-fat processed meats. They were promptly replaced with lean meats, fresh seafood, plentiful fresh fruits and vegetables, and a healthy smattering of nuts and seeds.

After eight weeks on this dietary regimen, Ethan began noticing a drastic change in his strength and endurance. He was lifting heavier, completing workouts faster, and had visible muscle mass gain. More importantly, he had lost 15 pounds. Ethan's story is a sterling example of how fine-tuning one's diet can lead to exceptional results in body composition and strength.

11.3. Serena's Swimming Success Story

Serena, a professional swimmer and coach, had always struggled with energy dips during her practice sessions. With the nature of her sport requiring sustained energy, this proved to be a significant challenge.

Consequently, Serena turned to the Paleo diet in the hopes of harnessing a more sustained form of energy. She swapped out bread, pasta, and dairy for fish, lean meats, vegetables, fruits, and nuts. Serena also invested in ensuring that her meals were a balance of protein, carbs, and good fats, all derived from Paleo-friendly sources.

The result was astonishing. Within six weeks, Serena found herself with increased energy and much fewer crashes during her training. Her performance in competitions improved tremendously, with her clocking in her personal best within the first three months of her dietary shift.

Given these riveting success stories, you too can chart your transformative journey in health and fitness. As seen from the experiences of Maya, Ethan, and Serena, the Paleo way of life can offer significant improvements in physical performance, recovery, and overall vitality. The path to peak performance doesn't lie in modern conveniences, rather harkens back to our ancestral nutritional wisdom. It's time to truly nourish our bodies and meet our fitness aspirations with the Paleo diet.

Chapter 12. The Paleo Performance Plan: Your Roadmap to Enhanced Fitness

In the realm of fitness and nutrition, harnessing the benefits of the ancient Paleo approach presents a compelling paradigm. The fidelity to a diet that our ancestors thrived upon aligns us to our genetic predispositions, providing untold benefits to our health and physical performance. This chapter details a structured plan creatively dubbed as 'The Paleo Performance Plan.' This comprehensive guide will walk you through a variety of actionable steps tailored towards infusing your body with the power of ancestral nutrition to elevate your fitness game.

12.1. Understanding Ancestral Nutrition

Let's start by understanding the premise behind the Paleo diet. At its core, it revolves around the notion that the closer we stick to the diet of our Paleolithic ancestors, the better our health, vitality, and athletic prowess become. Our ancestors were physically exceptional - they were lean, muscular, flexible, and hardy. The primary reason attributed to this is the type of food they consumed, which was devoid of processed, refined, and artificially produced items.

This essentially means favoring lean proteins, fruits, vegetables, seeds, nuts, and healthy fats, which were all readily available and consumed by our ancestors. On the opposite side, modern foods such as processed sugars, trans fats, and refined grains, which have been linked to various modern diseases and ailments, are excluded.

12.2. Creating Your Paleo Profile

Before jumping into any nutritional plan, it's crucial to understand that not all bodies work the same. We each have unique genetic predispositions, health histories, and lifestyle factors that influence how we respond to diet changes. Your Paleo profile will help tailor the general guidelines to your specific needs. Begin by assessing your overall health, activity levels, sensitivities, and goals. This could involve professional testing or simple self-observation.

12.3. Designing Your Paleo Plate

An effective Paleo plate should include a balance of high-quality proteins, a variety of non-starchy vegetables, healthy fats, minimal starchy vegetables or fruits, and absolutely no dairy, grains or processed foods.

Here's a breakdown of a typical Paleo plate:

- A fist-sized portion of lean protein (like lean meat, fish, or eggs)
- Two fistfuls of non-starchy vegetables
- A handful of nuts/seeds or healthful fats

Designing your Paleo plate this way ensures you're procuring a balance of macronutrients while simultaneously capitalizing on the micronutrient richness inherent in these food groups.

12.4. The Paleo Performance Hydration

Water was the main drink for our ancestors, but they also used to consume other fluids like bone broths which are rich in minerals. Hydration in the Paleo lifestyle would, therefore, include adequate clean water, alongside mineral-rich broths and, for those craving variety, unsweetened tea or black coffee.

12.5. Harmonizing Exercise with Paleo Diet

The caloric and nutritional needs of an athlete undertaking high-intensity workouts vary from those of an individual engaged in more moderate training. Depending on your training intensity and duration, you may need to adapt the diet.

If your training is of higher intensity or longer duration, you may need to increase your carbohydrate intake. This can be done by adding more starchy vegetables and fruits to your diet. Always ensure the adjustments are gradual and closely monitored for advantages and potential drawbacks.

12.6. Post-Workout Paleo Nutrition

Recovering from a workout involves the right balance of proteins and carbohydrates to restore muscle glycogen and to facilitate muscle repair and growth. Your post-workout Paleo plate should include a lean protein and a carbohydrate source like a starchy vegetable or fruit.

12.7. Conclusion

The Paleo Performance Plan extends beyond the realm of a 'diet.' It represents a change in lifestyle where you eat and live like your ancestors, thereby improving your health and fitness levels. The journey may be challenging and require discipline and dedication, but the reward is a wholesome body and an energized spirit ready for any physical tasks ahead.

Implement this comprehensive plan carefully, taking time to observe how your body responds to the changes. Remember, holistic wellbeing is the ultimate success in any fitness endeavor, and the Paleo performance plan, with its emphasis on natural foods and harmony with nature, aligns perfectly with this fundamental principle.